The
FLAT BELLY
MIRACLE

Access to
BONUS VIDEO
& OVER A DOZEN
Mouthwatering
Recipes!

EUGENE WALKER

How to Lose Belly Fat Fast & Get Your Sexy Back Forever!

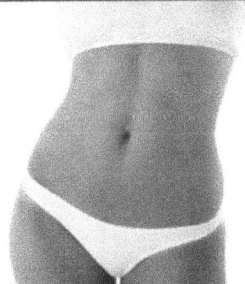
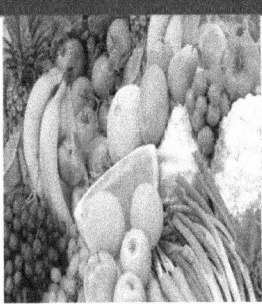
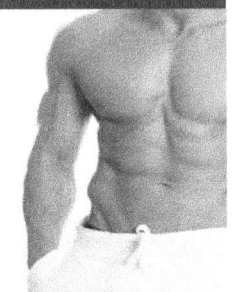

The information contained within **"The Flat Belly Miracle - How to Lose Belly Fat Fast and Get Your Sexy Back Forever"** is based on the author's own experience and research. The sources used for the research are credible and authentic to the best of our knowledge.

In no event shall the author be liable for any direct, indirect, incidental, punitive, or consequential damages of any kind whatsoever with respect to the service or the materials and the products contained within.

Table of Contents

Chapter 1 - Introduction

Chapter 2 - How to lose weight

Chapter 3 - How to set your goals

Chapter 4 - Macronutrients

Chapter 5 - Carbohydrates

Chapter 6 - Protein

Chapter 7 - Fats

Chapter 8 - Your Diet

Chapter 9 - Counting Calories

Chapter 10 - Low-Carb Diets

Chapter 11 - Paleo

Chapter 12 - The "Zone"

Chapter 13 - Misconceptions about weight loss

Chapter 14 - Women and Weight Training

Chapter 15 - "Toning" and Spot-reducing

Chapter 16 - Body Mass Index (BMI)

[Chapter 17 - Walking](#)

[Chapter 18 - Running](#)

[Chapter 19 - Cycling](#)

[Chapter 20 - P90X and Insanity](#)

[Chapter 21 - HHIT (High Intensity Interval Training)](#)

[Chapter 22 - Starting Strength](#)

[Chapter 23 - Strong Lifts 5X5](#)

[Chapter 24 - Cross fit](#)

[Chapter 25 - Cardio](#)

[Chapter 26 - Organized sports](#)

[Chapter 27 - Swimming](#)

[Chapter 28 - Zumba / Aerobics / Spinning / Yoga / Classes in general](#)

[Chapter 29 - How to deal with soreness after a workout](#)

[Chapter 30 - The importance of sleep](#)

[Chapter 31 - Supplements](#)

[Chapter 32 - Motivation](#)

[Chapter 33 - Things you'll notice as you're losing weight](#)

[Chapter 34 - Conclusion](#)

[Chapter 35 - ACCESS TO BONUS VIDEO AND RECIPES](#)

Chapter 1 - Introduction

Over the years, millions and millions of people, especially women, have struggled trying to lose belly fat. Whether it's to look better or be healthier, the fact is both men and women sometimes struggle to lose this weight. This in turn leads to frustration and eventually going back to the old way of doing things.

In this book I will try to address some of the most common dilemmas you may have come across when losing belly fat and how you can overcome them. We will review some of the most popular exercise regimes out there today and we will also review some of the most common dieting misconceptions that ultimately have lead some men and women to failure.

I hope you enjoy reading this book as much as I've enjoyed writing it and that my advice can help you reach your goals.

In this book you'll find several claims that have been researched and documented. However it is important to remember that I am not a doctor. If at any point you feel uncomfortable or concerned about any of the advice found in this book; please check with your physician first. This book is only to be taken as a very simplified-guide to weight loss and increased fitness with the aim of improving your overall health in the long term.

Some of the nutritional advice found in this book is meant for average people with no food allergies or special conditions. If you suffer from any of these please seek out professional advice before going on a diet.

Finally keep in mind that the power to lose weight is ultimately within you. As long as you stick to an exercise regime and watch what you eat I can guarantee that you'll succeed in your journey and as with millions of other people you'll reap the excellent benefits of improved health and fitness.

Chapter 2 - How to lose weight

Let me tell you one thing right off the bat, losing weight is not complicated, there is no "magic trick" or any ancient secrets to achieving your weight losing goals. Losing weight comes down to a very simple formula: -Eat fewer calories than you burn each day.

That's it! Simple, right? Yet many people, especially women think that they need to starve themselves or that they need to spend hours and hours at the gym every day in order to lose weight.

As long as you eat fewer calories than what your body needs, you WILL lose weight. I'm not saying this because I believe it's true, I'm saying this because it's a fact, backed by science, and it's a law of thermodynamics. As long as you keep your caloric intake below your BMR (more on this later) you will lose weight.

But how do you know how many calories your body needs and burns every day? You'll be surprised to know that you don't need to be a doctor or a dietician to figure this out. In order to calculate your BMR (Basal Metabolic Rate) this is; the amount of calories your body would burn if you stayed in bed all day, you use this simple formula:

BMR = 655 + (4.35 x weight in pounds) + (4.7 x height in inches) - (4.7 x age in years)

Let's take for example Carol, a 35 year old woman who is 5'5 tall and weighs 149 pounds. So that would be 655 + (4.35 x 149) + (4.7 x 65) – (4.7 x 35). That gives us 1445 calories per day. That's 1445 this person would need if she did nothing but sleep, however there's not too many people out there who sleep all day, Carol has an office job, which means that even though she doesn't move around a lot, she still has to walk to and from the parking lot, pickup groceries on the way home, and clean the house before she goes to bed.

By calculating her activity levels, we can assume that Carol burns an extra 350 calories every day just by doing her chores. On top of that, Carol goes to a yoga class 3 times per week, burning 300 calories per session. (You can use an online calculator to figure out how many calories you use up every day).

So let's add those numbers up. 1445 calories per day, times seven days a week gives us 10115 plus an extra 2450 calories per week from doing her chores plus 900 calories from 3 sessions of yoga per week for a grand total of 13465 calories per week, divided by 7 days which gives us a grand total of 1923 calories per day that Carol needs to MAINTAIN her current weight.

But Carol does not want to maintain! She wants to lose one pound per week, which is a healthy, reasonable weight loss. If you're really committed to your weight loss and want to accelerate things a bit you can aim for 2 pounds per week, but let's take it easy for now and stick with one pound per week.

A pound of fat is roughly equivalent to 3500 Calories. That means that if Carol wants to lose a pound of fat per week, she needs to eat 500 calories less per day, which gives us a total of 1423 calories per day if she keeps her activity levels the same.

Simple right? So what does carol need to do in order to eat at a deficit of 500 calories per day while feeling full? She needs to eat clean. More on "clean" eating later on.

 But for now the caloric needs of Carol have become very clear, see how it is not that complicated? In order to lose weight Carol will need to give up a few things in her life and become conscious of the decisions she takes. Is it really worth it to eat that Snickers bar that has 40 grams of fat and 600 calories?

Wouldn't you rather eat something that is filling, tasty and healthy? 600 calories is a lot! Some people don't even eat that much for breakfast. Yet if you eat that chocolate bar you won't even feel full, you'll feel full of regrets perhaps but that's it. You'll be hungry again in 2 hours and you'll have to shove down another 600 calories down your throat like it's no problem.

Sorry for the rant there but it is a very common mistake that I see with newbies every day. Do not fool yourself into thinking you're eating healthy if you're not. And do not set unrealistic goals for yourself.

Chapter 3 - How to set your goals

The very first thing you need to do before you begin a regime is to know where you're at and where you want to go. From now on, every day when you wake up, the first thing you will do is weight yourself. Before you go eat or drink anything, before you do any activities, before you even go to the bathroom! You must weight yourself as accurately as possible.

Strip down to your underwear and step into the scale (If you have access to an iron-beam scale these are more accurate than your traditional bathroom scales). Once you've weighted yourself you're going to measure yourself. Measure your breast line right above the nipple, measure your hips right at the top of your hip bones and measure your waist, about half an inch above the belly button.

Once you've got all these numbers down, you're going to write these down in your journal. I don't care if it's an online journal, your cell phone, an actual notebook or a post-it note. You must do this every day until you have reached your goals.

In order to know where you want to go we have to take some factors into consideration. Do you want to simply lose fat or do you want to build muscle? Truth is most women do not want to build muscle as they think they will get "bulky" or "manly".

This is a LIE, unless you start eating like a champ (I'm talking 3000 calories per day or more) and get into some serious supplement (legal or otherwise) usage. You won't end up looking like the she-Hulk. However, you should know that if your intention is to build muscle, this book is not for you.

In order to gain muscle you have to gain weight and have a very tight control over your macronutrients in order to eat at a calorie surplus. Since we will teach you how to eat at deficit in this book, it will be very difficult if not possible to achieve your muscle-gaining goals.

But you don't want to build muscle, you want to lose fat. In order to lose fat we've already established that we have to eat at a deficit, that deficit for carol is about 500 calories per day until she reaches her desired weight. But how will Carol know what her desired weight is? A very common formula to calculate someone's desired weight is:

53.1 kg + 1.36 kg per inch over 5 feet

This gives us a figure of around 135 pounds for Carol's ideal weight. Since she is 149 pounds right now, she will need to lose 14 pounds in order to reach her ideal weight. Keep in mind that once you start to lose weight you will need to recalculate your caloric intake and needs every week.

This means that in about 14 weeks or 3 and a half months Carol will lose those 14 pounds in a healthy, safe way. Without risking her health or the impending risk of yo-yoing after she has reached her ideal weight.

These are the very basics of weight loss, other than that it is important to keep your goals realistic, first off if you want to lose 10 pounds by your best friend's wedding in 2 weeks, I can tell you right now that it isn't happening.

Weight loss is a long journey and you must make small sacrifices that will help you ultimately reach your weight losing goals. Possibly the most difficult realization that will face is the fact that your lifestyle needs to change.

You will not go on a diet; you will CHANGE your diet. If you revert to your old habits, your body will too revert to its old weight. Always strive to improve yourself and to better yourself. These changes will take time, and a bit of sacrifice, but if you're willing to improve yourself nothing can stop you.

Once you've decided what you want to achieve; both in the long term and in the short term, you need to create a plan to achieve these goals. Let's go back for a second to that magic number we came up with a few pages ago, that magic number that will help you reach your goals; your caloric deficit.

Once you've got this deficit figured out, how you want to get to it every day depends entirely on you. You can either change your feeding habits or do more exercise. Ideally you want a combination of both so that the changes don't feel so drastic.

Remember though, how you want to achieve this basic aim of consuming less calories than what your body needs will depend entirely on you, your lifestyle, your habits, your preferences and your long term and short term goals.

The most important thing to remember is to be patient and not to get discouraged. Losing weight takes time and sometimes progress can slow down. If you're getting discouraged by how slowly you're losing weight think about how long it took you to put on that weight.

Chapter 4 - Macronutrients

When you're trying to figure out what diet to go on you will notice that online and in many books, authors use the term "Macronutrients" or "Macros" to refer to certain nutrients in general. Macronutrients are one of 3 (technically 4 as alcohol is a macro as well) nutrients that provide energy to the body.

These macronutrients are needed to sustain the vital functions in the body such as growth, metabolism, repair and more. There are three basic macronutrients' Carbohydrates, Fat and Protein. A gram of carbohydrates gives the body 4 calories per gram.

Protein will provide the body with 4 calories per gram and fat provides 9 calories per gram. Looking at a nutritional label if you're eating something that has 10 grams of carbs, 5 grams of protein and 5 grams of fat you can easily calculate the total calories this food will provide. 10 grams of carbs equals 40 calories, 5 grams of protein equals 20 calories and 5 grams of fat equals 45 calories, giving us a total of 105 calories per portion.

Let's take a quick look at each macronutrient.

Chapter 5 - Carbohydrates

Carbs are a large molecule that consist of carbon, hydrogen and oxygen and usually divided in 4 major categories: monosaccharaides, disaccharides, oligosaccharides, and polysaccharides. Generally speaking the first two are referred to as sugars. Things like honey, refined sugar, cane sugar, glucose, lactose and more.

Carbs play a very important role in the human body. Carbs are usually stored as energy by the human body (mainly starch and glycogen) and are also used as structural components. Carbs are used by the body as the main source of fuel and are the first source of energy the body goes to when looking for energy.

Carbs are also very important for our body and the central nervous system as well as the brain, the muscles and the kidney to function properly and are usually found in starchy foods like cereals, grains, potatoes, fruit, some vegetables, dairy and pasta.

It is possible that you might hear that excess carbohydrates are bad. I do not necessarily think they are bad for you but I do think that limiting the amount of carbohydrates in your diet is always a good idea. Aim for carbs that are high in fiber, go for whole wheat pastas and brown rice.

Yams and red potatoes are good too as they will provide the energy you need to fuel through your day but are also very rich in fiber which helps the digestive system function properly and it aids digestion as well. Fiber cannot be digested by our GI so these carbs simply pass through the intestinal tract intact and help your body get rid of the waste.

When calculating your carbs for low-carbs diets keep in mind to subtract the amount of carbs you get from fiber towards your total carb count. Diets that are low in fiber have been shown to cause intestinal problems such as constipation and hemorrhoids and have been show to create more problems down the road. If you decide to go on a low carb diet make sure to ingest fiber supplements in order to maintain regular bowel movements.

Chapter 6 - Protein

When we consume foods with protein in them, our body starts to break down the protein into building blocks called amino acids. Some amino acids are vital to the human body and we MUST get them from our diet and some amino acids are non-vital which means the body will produce them on demand. Protein rich foods include all types of meat; beef, poultry, fish, seafood, veal, buffalo, ostrich, turkey, etc. Eggs, milk, seeds, nuts, cheese, yogurt, some cereals, some vegetables and some fruit also contain considerable amounts of protein.

Protein is used by our body to promote growth and it is hugely important for children, teens, pregnant women and bodybuilders. If you are trying to get big muscles you must consume at least 1 gram of protein per pound of body mass.

Protein also aids in tissue repair and it strengthens the immune system by producing essential hormones and enzymes. Once the amount of carbs in your body is low and the body requires more energy, the body will start converting excess protein into carbs.

Finally, if you're already a big bodybuilder and you want to stay that way, it is important that you consume enough protein. The good news is that most Americans get more than enough protein from their diet.

If you feel like you are not getting enough food from your diet a good thing to consider is whey protein, a natural protein found in dairy that is sold over the counter and has become extremely popular in recent years for its low cost and easy availability.

Keep in mind that whey does not have any special properties and it won't magically help you grow muscle. It is simply a supplement for people who cannot get enough protein into their diet from other sources.

If you're a vegetarian you have plenty of options when it comes to getting protein in your diet, things like beans, lentils, chia seeds and some vegetables are packed with protein! There's also vegetarian whey protein out there in case you don't want to struggle.

Chapter 7 - Fats

Ah yes, fats. You've probably heard about how all fats are bad and how fats will kill you and that anything that is low-fat automatically becomes super healthy. But this couldn't be further from the truth. Fats have gained a bad reputation for causing weight gains but fats are essential for some body functions.

In fact our bodies can survive without eating any carbs at all but you'd still need to eat fats. Fats in our body are used for energy as it is the most concentrated source of energy, it is also essential for growth and development and it plays a vital role in the absorption of certain vitamins.

Fat can be found in a variety of foods that include meats, milk, nuts, and some vegetables and fruits as avocado and coconut (both excellent sources of good fats).

But what exactly are good fats and bad fats? Bad fats are usually Trans and saturated fats found in foods because they bring up your cholesterol level and increase your risk for heart disease.

Foods rich in Tran's fat are things like: French fries, pies, anything that is deep fried or battered, margarine, shortening, lard, cakes, frosting, fried chicken, ice cream, cookies, biscuits, etcetera.

See a pattern here? It is generally a good idea to avoid fats such as lard and shortening and things that are deep fried. Not that difficult right? But what about the good fats? Good fats are those in the group of monosaturated fats and polyunsaturated fats.

These will lower your cholesterol levels and reduce your risk of heart disease. Foods rich in good fats are flaxseed oil, butter, coconut oil, avocado, soybean, dairies, nuts, seeds, chocolate (yes, dark, bitter chocolate) and more.

It is important to keep a balance between these two different types of fats in order to avoid the complications that an excess of fats will bring in the future.

Keep in mind that lowering the amount of fads you consume is not the most important thing, it is more important to keep a good balance of fats that you eat rather than focusing on the total amount of fats in your diet. A good balance of fats will ensure your cholesterol levels stay down.

For many decades, several doctors, dietitians and health authorities have told us that a diet that is rich in saturated fats will raise blood cholesterol levels and increase the risk of heart disease such as cardiac arrests and strokes.

However, recent studies have proven that people who eat lots of saturated fat do not put themselves at a higher risk of disease that those who don't. HOWEVER, this does not mean you should go all out on saturated fats. It is important to learn how to make healthy substitutions when it comes to saturated fats.

For example switching out animal fats for vegetable fats will go a long way towards improving your overall health. To put it simply, nothing has changed. Reducing the amount of saturated fats in your diet will definitely improve your heart health as long as you replace it with good fat and not simple carbs or refined sugars.

Finally, eating a low-fat diet does not mean you'll stay thin forever. If you stuff yourself with simple carbs and sugars you'll still struggle to lose weight. Obesity rates for Americans have almost doubled in the last 20 years which is when the whole low-fat craze started.

Rather than focusing on eating low-fat, it is more important to focus on maintaining a good ratio of macronutrients in your body.

But what ratio is the "right" ratio of macros? It depends on who you ask. If you ask someone who is doing a low carb diet they will tell you something along the lines of 10% or less carbs, 45% protein and 45% fat. If you ask someone who's doing a high protein, low fat diet, they'll tell you, 25-50-25.

Ask a calorie zone dieter and he will tell you 40-40-20. The truth is that whatever plans you decide to go on, you need to analyze your goals and your timeframe before you decide what diet to go on. Do you want to build a lot of lean mass?

Try a high protein diet. Do you want to drop fat QUICKLY? Try a low carb diet. Do you want to improve your overall appearance without making too many drastic changes? Maybe the Zone works for you.

I went ahead and did a bit of research on the most popular diets nowadays so that you may decide which one works for you. This is by no means a definitive guide and you may follow other programs as you wish. Make sure to check with your physician first before you embark into a diet or fitness program.

Chapter 8 - Your Diet

As we mentioned before, diet is the most vital part of losing weight for most people, watching what you eat is very important step in reaching your goals. There are two simple approaches that people usually take when starting out; they can ease into it by making small changes one step at a time, such as cutting out sugar or alcohol or to completely change overnight.

Whichever way you decided to go, keep in mind that both approaches are just fine. Go with what makes you feel comfortable; however there are many diets out there that can help you achieve your goals faster. Let's take some time and discuss some of the most popular diets out there.

Chapter 9 - Counting Calories

The most popular diet by far. In this diet you write down EVERY SINGLE THING that you eat and how much of it you ate (I recommend getting a small food scale). And then write it down in a journal or a calorie-tracking app. (I recommend myfitnesspal). The basic idea is to ultimately eat fewer calories than what your body needs.

What your body fails to get from food it will get from your fat reserves, thus burning body fat. If you're aiming for a specific caloric intake it is very important to make those calories count. Could you eat 1445 calories of candy a day and still lose weight? Well, yes.

But it is going to make you feel miserable because you're going to be hungry all the time and you're not going to have any energy to do your everyday tasks. This is where the concept of "Eating Clean" comes in. Eating foods that will make you feel full and give you the energy that you need every day; I'm talking foods that are high in protein or fiber and low in fat.

Things like Chicken breast, turkey meat, steaks, tuna, lean ground beef, fish, nuts, berries, green vegetables, eggs, lean cold cuts, whole wheat pasta, milk, brown rice and a little bit of fruit are examples of food that not only is low on calories but also filling and good in nutrients.

If you decide to start counting calories it is very important that you make every calorie count. Do not eat empty calories full of sugar and carbs that will have you feeling hungry again in 2 hours. Eat foods high in fiber and high in protein. These foods will not only have you feeling full for most of the day but they will also make you healthier in the long run.

You might've heard this before "A calorie is a calorie, regardless of where it comes from" I can tell you that while technically true, it does not mean what you think it means. Can you eat nothing but 1600 calories of candy a day and still lose weight? Technically yes but you'll feel miserable and hate yourself after a day or two and we do not want that.

We want you to feel full and healthy, with enough energy to do the things that you need to do and we want you to feel satisfied. One of the most common reasons why people abandon their diets is because they eat like crap and end up feeling like crap. You won't survive by eating salads all day. You need protein and carbs to help you get through the day. Keep this in mind when choosing a diet.

Chapter 10 - Low-Carb Diets

Low carb diets have become very popular over the last 15 years or so due to the fact that they offer a lot of options and follow a very basic premise. Low-carb diets work on the basis that carbs are converted to sugar very rapidly, causing your body to feel hungry and causing a reaction that triggers your body to store fat. Obviously all carbs that don't come from fiber are a huge no-no in low-carb diets, things like sugar, dairy, flour; pasta and bread are not allowed at all.

Chapter 11 - Paleo

Paleo is one of the most popular diets nowadays and it seems to keep getting more and more popular every day. According to Paleo followers, it is a great way to get healthier and lose weight naturally while improving other aspects of your life.

Paleo is a natural nutritional approach that works together with your genetics in order to help you put off weight and stay lean by building a healthy diet with protein as the main source of calories and it aims to copy the feeding habits of our Paleolithic ancestors (thus the name Paleo).

Some of the foods that are okay to eat in Paleo are lean meats, seafood, nuts, berries, seeds, vegetables, fruit and healthy fats such as coconut and avocado oil. Paleo seems to work for a lot of people and will give you healthy benefits such as stable blood sugar levels, clear skin, better teeth, and improved sleep and reduced allergies.

Chapter 12 - The "Zone"

This is another diet that focuses on the quality of the food rather than quantity. It focuses on balancing the percentages of "macros" (Macronutrients, protein, fat and carbs) while providing a hormonal balance that will help you burn fat off.

I would say this is one of the harder diets to follow because you will most likely need to track down and write down everything that you eat, but I can guarantee that being strict about it will pay off in the long run. I have to admit that I have not personally tried this diet myself but I have heard great things about it especially from high-performance athletes and bodybuilders who swear by it.

The truth about fad diets, cleanses, 24 hour diets, etc.

Please do not fool yourself into thinking any of these fast weight losing methods will work. Losing weight is a long journey that requires effort and sacrifice. Fooling yourself into thinking that a Kiwi-Pineapple smoothie or massive amounts of cabbage soup will make you lose weight will lead to nothing but disappointment and frustration in the long run. Yes, you may lose a pound here and there but you will put it back immediately after you go back to your old habits.

"Cleanses" do absolutely nothing for you either, the only thing cleanses do is flush out the electrolytes that your body needs and as soon as you replace them the weight will come back. Besides, ingesting large amounts of sugary drinks (even if they come from fruit) is never a good idea. In short, none of these work and they won't provide the long-term results you're looking for.

Here's a list of fad diets that you should not waste your time with:

Acai Berry, 3-Day Diet, Cabbage soup, Negative calorie diet, Hollywood diet, Apple Cider Vinegar diet, Beverly Hills Diet, Grapefruit diet.

And as always, remember that if it sounds too good to be true, then it probably is.

Chapter 13 - Misconceptions about weight loss

One of the main issues that people come across when losing weight is the huge amount of information that is found on different sources. And unfortunately some of it ends up not being true or highly exaggerated. Let's go over some of the most common misconceptions people have.

Chapter 14 - Women and Weight Training

This one is very common and it makes me really confused. Some women will avoid weight training or weight lifting for fear or gaining more muscle than what they want and they're afraid they will end up looking bulky, manly or huge.

Let's talk about the chemistry of muscle-building first. When you lift weights, you create microscopic tears in your muscle, once your body detects this, it starts pumping fluids (mainly water) into your muscles in order to repair that muscle. This process is aided by amino acids in your body that come from protein sources and aided by some hormones as well (mainly testosterone).

As a woman, the only way you're going to end up looking like those women in bodybuilding contests is by either consuming massive amounts of protein or getting testosterone injections. Well, that or using steroids. If you lift weights the only thing that will happen is that you will continue losing fat and getting leaner and stronger. Even men with high levels of testosterone will struggle gaining more than a pound of lean muscle a month.

Chapter 15 - "Toning" and Spot-reducing

HUGE fallacies right here. Let's go over toning first. You may have heard this at the gym "Lift high-weight and low-rep" for strength and "low weight, high rep for toning". Toning up is a meaningless term, it simply means having a defined body which will come from two things, Losing fat and building muscle. You can't get "tone definition" unless you burn some fat off your body.

Spot reducing on the other hand is physically impossible. It's natural that you might want to lose fat in certain areas of your body like your stomach, your thighs or your arms, unfortunately it is impossible to spot reduce fat in your body. You can do all the crunches you want in the morning, but unless you change the way you eat and lose weight overall those love handles aren't going anywhere.

Chapter 16 - Body Mass Index (BMI)

BMI is a number that is calculated using your height and weight. It is, however a very inaccurate way of determining someone's health. It should only be considered a very rough guide and it is not by any means an indication of health. Keep in mind that a6'3 bodybuilder with 6% body fat who is 250 pounds has the same BMI as an overweight man who is the same height.

BMI is only meant to be used as a very rough reference and should never be used to determine your weight-loss goals.

Is it possible to lose fat and gain mass at the same time?

One of the most common misconceptions people have when it comes to losing weight and getting fitter is that it is impossible to gain muscle while losing fat. You have to choose and settle for one of those two; however this is nothing but a huge misconception, It IS possible to do both at the same time and the ability to gain muscle while losing fat is entirely dependent on the relationship between your fat body percentage and muscularity.

An obese, under-trained person will be able to lose fat and gain muscle at the same time during the first 3-4 months of weight training due to a Central Nervous System response and thus it will be very simple for this person to achieve both at the same time. However, a person who is very lean and near his lean mass building limits will struggle to gain mass.

Once you have attained decent mass gains the only way to achieve fat loss without losing mass is to continue eating at a slight caloric deficit while consuming at least a gram of protein per pound of mass. For example if you're a 180 pound lifter then you will need to eat at least 180 grams of protein a day, while maintaining a slight caloric deficit.

Since achieving this balance for most people is extremely difficult, most people who are trying to get leaner will go into of one two cycles known as "bulking" and "cutting". Let's take a quick look at both of them.

It is very possible that you may have already hear these terms before, possibly in weight loss magazines, or bodybuilding forums, websites or whatever. Should you do this?

The answer is; unless you are a very serious bodybuilder or professional lifter then no, because these are the only 2 groups who will benefit from bulking and cutting. Beginner and intermediates will not benefit from this as weight swings are not good for your body. It is also important to learn how maintain a healthy diet that not only helps you achieve the results you want but also makes you enjoy the food you're eating.

Exercise regimes

Let's go over some of the most exercise regimes that are available to those with access to a gym and those without access to a gym.

For those without access to a gym

Chapter 17 - Walking

Let me get this off my chest. I don't consider walking to be a true workout. Going for a stroll in the park or walking your dog will give you a very small caloric deficit that might not even be worth your time. If you want to take up walking as your exercise regime you need to make it worth your time; carry a heavy bag with you, walk up an incline road, power walk or hike.

Chapter 18 - Running

One of the most popular workouts in the world since it requires almost no equipment (other than a good pair of running shoes). One of the most popular programs that involve running is Couch to 5K, a program that will take you from couch potato to running a full 5k in 9 weeks. It is very simple to follow and it does a great job scaling your runs so you don't exhaust yourself.

The program has already worked for hundreds of thousands of people and I personally did it about 5 years ago. Make sure you take some music with your and enjoy the scenery out there. If the weather doesn't allow it you might consider training in a treadmill.

Chapter 19 - Cycling

Another massively popular workout that requires a bit more of equipment, mainly a good bike and a helmet. It is a great opportunity to see the great outdoors while getting fit. I can't talk too much about Cycling because I've never practiced it at that level but you can't find plenty of info online and in forums.

Chapter 20 - P90X and Insanity

Two very popular home workout routines that do require a bit of equipment (mainly a pull-up bar and two dumbbells). Keep in mind that these 2 programs are aimed towards beginners and you will probably hit a plateau sooner or later, however as starting conditioning programs I think they're fantastic.

Calisthenics and bodyweight training.

Things that you can do with your own weight, like pushups, jumping jacks, crunches, squats, planks, etc. There are several programs out there like simple fit and convict conditioning. Look them up if you're interested in doing this at home. Keep in mind that if you're overweight at first you might struggle with this when beginning.

Chapter 21 - HHIT (High Intensity Interval Training)

Short burst of various exercises over an extended period of time (For example sprinting for a minute, and then doing 10 pushups, followed by 10 squats, resting for 90 seconds and repeating). Very effective for weight loss and improved health overall. Almost no required equipment is necessary and it is good for both beginning and experienced athletes.

8-minute-abs, 5 minutes a day, infomercials, etc.

None of these actually do anything for your help or help you lose weight. Any abs programs that promise to deliver results by working out a few minutes a day are nothing but lies. First off people who have visible abs do it by bringing their fat body percentages around or below 14%. You can do a million crunches a day, but if you got a huge beer belly then it is all going to be pointless since you'll never see abs until you drop those fat pounds.

And then there are programs that promise to deliver great health benefits by working out 5 or 10 minutes a day. Again, lies. Unless it is very, VERY high intensity training then it probably won't do anything for you. Remember if you want to see results then you really have to sweat it out there.

For those with access to a gym

Chapter 22 - Starting Strength

Starting Strength (or SS) is a weightlifting program designed by Mark Rippetoe designed to provide a solid foundation for weightlifting and strength gains in a short to medium time range. Even though it requires a bit of equipment (Mainly a barbell, some plates and a squat rack) you should be able to find these at any decent gym.

Keep in mind that even though this program is mainly aimed towards men who will see gains quicker due the high-testosterone levels it is still a useful program for women as it will proved a solid foundation for more technical lifts.

Starting strength is an excellent book for learning proper techniques for learning barbell lifts such as the dead lift, the bench press and the power clean. The program, however does have its fair share of criticism as one of the claims Rippetoe makes in its book is the fact that a person can expect to gain over 30 pounds of lean mass in 11 weeks and this is nothing but lies, as we mentioned before even a person with high levels of testosterone and perfect nutrition won't achieve these results IN A YEAR, let alone 11 weeks.

The nutritional advice given by Rippetoe is also sketchy at best. Don't get me wrong, doing a clean bulk is fine, but eating 5000 calories a day serves absolutely no purpose at all. If you follow Rippetoe's advice you'll end up strong, sure. But you'll end up very fat.

The verdict: Use it to learn proper technique and form ignore the nutritional advice.

Chapter 23 - Strong Lifts 5X5

Strong lifts is another strength building program built on the 5X5 principle in which you do each exercise for five sets of five repetitions. Each repetition is done at the same weight for all sets and you add weight each workout until you hit your PR. Even though no one knows exactly where this program came from, most people attribute its popularization to champion lifter and famous coach Bill Starr. This program has two workout routines which are then alternated.

The first routine includes the back squat, the bench press and the barbell rows, while the second program includes the back squat, the overhead press and the dead lift.

Not only will this program help you achieve decent gains but as with SS it is a great foundation for technical lifts, However it is very easy to reach a plateau and sooner or later your gains will plateau as well, it is recommended that you do this program for 9 months at the most and then switch to a more specific routine designed by a coach.

The verdict: Very good for beginners, not so much for intermediate to advanced lifters.

Chapter 24 - Cross fit

Cross fit is a cross-training program designed by Greg Glassman that focuses on building functional strength and HIIT (High Intensity Interval Training); it aims to train people on all aspects of fitness (strength, flexibility and endurance) by mixing all these elements into a workout.

Cross fit offers excellent stability, making it perfect for beginners as well as experts as it scales loads and intensities without changing the programming. Cross fit has gained a lot of popularity in recent years but it has also generated a lot of criticism due to its cult-like mentality and some irresponsible trainers who focus on the number of reps rather than good form.

When done correctly though, cross fit is an excellent way to achieve fitness while having fun and no matter where you live it should be fairly easy to find a gym (or box, as they call gyms) to train at.

The verdict: Do your research before joining a box.

Chapter 25 - Cardio

Cardio is an excellent way to lose fat (you won't gain any muscle though) and gyms are PACKED with cardio machines. At any decent gym you should be able to find treadmills, elliptical machines, escalators, stationary bikes and more.

While I always recommend doing a bit of cardio with every workout it is important to be wary of the claims made by calorie counters on cardio machines and to also watch out for potential injuries as cardio machines have some of the highest rates of injuries for starting athletes.

If you're obese or severely overweight consider training on the elliptical machine or stationery bike instead of the treadmill in order to reduce the impact to your knees and ankles.

The verdict: Good for weight loss, be wary of injuries.

Chapter 26 - Organized sports

Organized Sports is an excellent way to get fit while getting to know new people. Whether it is something light like tennis or badminton or something really demanding like American football or Ice hockey you'll find yourself having a lot of fun and burning a crazy amount of calories, sometimes without even noticing!

Since sports are obviously very competitive, if you're not very good at a sport yet, try to find a sport where people do it simply for fun, like a Sunday league or intramural sports.

The verdict: Good for organized fun, avoid overly-competitive leagues.

Chapter 27 - Swimming

Some people believe swimming is one of the best workouts you can ever take on. You'll exercise nearly every muscle in your body while improving your endurance and cardio ability.

If you can find a gym with a built in pool then by all means give it a try. Be aware though! Some people can find swimming to be extremely dull and boring but some people will swear by it. If you have access to a pool then by all means give it a try.

The verdict: Excellent all-around workout. Can be a bit boring though.

Chapter 28 - Zumba / Aerobics / Spinning / Yoga / Classes in general

These can be very fun and you will generally find yourself surrounded by a supportive community that will have the same goals as you do, there are a million different classes out there so I won't go into any specifics but I have taken a few and can say for sure that I always found myself getting a good workout and had a lot of fun.

Try a few different classes out and stick with the one you like. If you end up liking a few different classes then by all means go to as many as you can! Come up with your own programming and decide on what you want to get out of each class. Commit to your program and as with all the other regimes described in this book make sure you track your progress so that you don't get discouraged.

The verdict: Can be a lot of fun and you'll always get a good workout. Can be difficult who people who are intimidated by large crowds or coaches in general.

Chapter 29 - How to deal with soreness after a workout

We all know the feeling, you haven't worked out in a few weeks/months/years and the first day after you go back to the gym for the first time you're barely able to move. Your whole body aches like you've just been run over by a trailer and getting out of bed does not seem like an option.

What you're experiencing is called DOMS or Delayed on-set muscle soreness. In order to understand how to treat DOMS we need to understand first what causes it.

DOMS (also known as muscle fever) is what we call the pain and general feel of stiffness in our muscles that we get a few hours after unaccustomed exercise. DOMS is felt more strongly 24 hours after the exercise and it is caused by minor trauma to the muscle, basically what happens is that micro-tears in your muscle are trying to heal up by pumping several chemical compounds into your muscle.

If you continue exercising regularly the body will quickly adapt to these changes and you won't get DOMS anymore.

Keep in mind though that even though DOMS is a symptom usually associated with muscle damage, it does not necessarily mean that you have damaged your muscles. The soreness will come exclusively from temporary changes caused in muscles by exercise.

DOMS does not care whether you're young or old, male or female. DOMS does not discriminate end everyone can and will get DOMS. Even though it is almost impossible to prevent it, there are some things we can do to reduce the pain in order to be able to work out again.

People back in the day used to think that DOMS and recovery could be sped up by increasing the amount of food that we ate. It is now clear; however that while repairing structural damage to muscles is quite simple.

One of the best solutions for DOMS is to use enzymes that accelerate the healing process in the body such as protease and sitosterols. Protease enzymes are essential because they play a vital role in the inflammatory process that precedes

DOMS. While Sistosterols are plant-based enzymes that reduce cortisol in the body and have a direct muscle-building effect.

By consuming non-steroidal anti-inflammatory drugs (NSAID's) you may also help relieve pain caused by DOMS, drugs like aspirin and ibuprofen may help relieve pain, try to reduce the intake of these drugs however, as some recent studies have proven that NSAIDs have an indirect effect in reducing lean muscle gains.

It is also important to know how to respect your limits and to be aware of your limitations at the gym. Don't expect to go in the first day, being able to dead lift 300 pounds without there being any consequences.

As always, remember to do a full body stretch routine before you get into any serious exercise. One of the best ways to deal with DOMS in my opinion is to get a foam roller and learn some basic rolls so that you can heal faster.

But what is a foam roller? If this is the first time you've heard of this term, I'll clear it up for you. A foam roller is a versatile piece of equipment made out of foam that is used for self myofascial release.

Self Myofascial Release is another term for self-massage that aims to improve muscle flexibility by applying pressure to specific points on your body, thus improving your flexibility, elasticity and overall muscle health.

Even though this technique has gained a lot of popularity in recent times, it used to be a mysterious technique used only by professionals in different industries but it has now grown into a widely-popular technique that is used by athletes of all levels.

By targeting known "trigger points" also known as knots that form in our muscles foam rolling aims to relieve pressure in our muscles by "untying" these knots. An example of these "knots" that form in our bodies is felt when rolling your IT band which causes pain to extend all the way down to the leg or ankle.

Think of it as the kind of pain you get when doing stretches, it is supposed to hurt a little bit but not to be unbearable. As always check with your physician before going all-out with the roller or any of the advice given in this book.

Chapter 30 - The importance of sleep

If you're like the majority of American adults, it is quite likely that you do not get enough sleep every day to fully recover after a workout. Believe it or not, it is possible that your lack of proper sleep could be causing you to gain weight.

Instead of focusing on getting a good night's sleep we focus on getting our energy from a cup of coffee or sugary treats which ultimately leads to weight gain. This also means that since you're tired you won't likely have time to cook a healthy meal, so you'll go for some fast food after work and end up eating a million calories.

It is a vicious cycle that ultimately leads to less activity levels and more caloric intake. It is natural for our brains to respond to the lack of sleep by going for comfort foods. But what is the immediate result of this? Yes, you'll be able to stay awake but at what cost? Unwanted fat, lessened gains, bad mood, tiredness, irritability, and other symptoms.

One of the most important side effects of sleep deprivation is slowed down metabolism. I'm sure you've heard this term before but what exactly is metabolism?

According to Wikipedia, metabolism is the set of life sustaining chemical transformations within the cells of living organisms. What this means for is that metabolism is the process by which your body converts food into energy (remember? Calories in and calories out?)

If food is quickly absorbed by the organism and converted into energy the chances of it becoming fat reserves is almost null. But people with slow metabolisms will have a harder time turning food into energy. And whatever energy doesn't end up being used will end up being stored away as fat.

Going back to the topic of sleep, sleep also plays a vital role in mass building. See, when our muscles suffer micro tears after a workout, the system starts pumping fluids into the muscle in order to repair the muscle and make it denser. This process has it most vital functions linked to sleep as most of the repairs are done when we sleep.

But what happens if you don't get enough sleep? Then the process will be cut short and you'll be missing out on some sweet gains. Remember that sleep is like a credit card, if you keep accumulating debt then your body will crash.

The recommended amount of sleep a human adult should get fluctuates between seven and eight hours depending on a few different factors such as levels of activity, your daily routine and nutrition. You should be aiming for at least 8 hours every day.

I know it sounds difficult and it may sound like you won't have enough time to do your chores everyday but believe me, you cannot afford to sacrifice hours of sleep in order to get other stuff done. When it comes to your health the amount of sleep you get will determine how your body will react to different situations such as illness, injury or anxiety so it is hugely important that you get your 8 hours every day.

But what can you do about sleep deprivation? First of all you have to take a look and make an analysis on how much you sleep and how well you sleep. It doesn't matter if you sleep 8 hours a day if you keep waking up every 2 hours because it's too hot or because you need to pee.

Ideally you should be getting 8 continuous hours of sleep every day. If you need to get up for whatever reason then it is acceptable to break up your sleep periods in 2 periods of 4 hours each. Any shorter than that and you'll be severely affecting the quality of your sleep.

A good tip to keep in mind is to avoid caffeine after noon. Studies have shown that high intakes of caffeine after noon decrease the quality and quantity of your sleep. Do a bit of exercise before bed.

If you do your heavy workouts in the morning then do a bit of yoga before bed or a bit of light stretching. Nothing too strenuous as we don't want your body to go into a full caloric burn.

Watch what you eat before bed. Avoid eating big meals at least 4 hours before bedtime and avoid simple carbohydrates and foods high in sugar. If you eat any of these foods you will make it more difficult for your body to go into a state of deep-sleep.

A glass of liquor or one beer is ok before bed every once in a while, but don't let it become a crutch and watch out for those empty calories. Think of it as it being a treat rather than something that you deserve.

If for any reason you still feel sleepy after getting a continuous 8 hours of sleep then it might be a good idea to speak to your doctor. There are several reasons why your body could be demanding more sleep.

Things like high-stress work environments, bad nutrition, or maybe you're pushing yourself too hard at the gym. Keep in mind that you'll need to listen to your body in order to try to improve its condition. If everything else fails you can get a deep-sleep study done so that the causes behind your lack of rest can be determined.

In a deep sleep study you are monitored while sleeping so that the sleep specialist can determine the cause of your problems and so that he can identify the root cause of the issue.

Remember that by providing our body with the nutrients and the rest it needs we are creating an ideal environment for weight loss and muscle gains. Don't waste all your efforts just because you don't want to go to bed early.

One last thing. When you go to sleep, go to sleep. Don't bring your laptop with you. Leave your Smartphone away and concentrate and prepare yourself to go to sleep. A bit of light reading is fine but try not to distract yourself too much from your main goal which is sleeping.

Remember to create an ideal environment for your night's sleep. Make sure your pillows are comfy and your sheets are clean, leave the thermostat at an ideal temperature and make sure your rooms is free of any distracting sounds and that it is clean as well.

Chapter 31 - Supplements

I know I know you might've heard about how dieting supplements are dangerous for you and how they will get your heart racing and how you'll eventually end with a heart attack or a bad live.

Truth is, there are thousands of supplements available out there and as long as you know what you're consuming and what the advantages and disadvantage of each supplement are you should be ok. In this book we will be reviewing only legal supplements that will help you achieve the goals you want.

I have no interest, nor have I ever tried any illegal supplements and I don't want you to use them either. Obviously supplements are not necessary for weight loss but if you can afford to buy them I can't see them doing any harm.

Green Tea Extract

Green tea extract is a supplement that is proven to work as it contains antioxidant ingredients such as catechins that comprise four major epicatechin derivatives as well as flavonoids and caffeine. Green tea extract is proven to contain more antioxidant properties than vitamin C. Green tea extract also contains anti-carcinogen, anti-radiation and anti-inflammatory properties.

Calcium

Calcium is a mineral found in several foods such as dairies and works alongside vitamin D to provide the nutrients necessary to create a healthy fat-burning environment. Calcium is normally stored in fat cells and recent studies have found out that the more calcium a fat cell has the more fat that cell will burn in the long term. Calcium also helps reduce the rate of absorption of fat in the GI tract, reducing the amount of excess fat your body will store from fatty foods.

Whey Protein

Excellent supplement for people who are trying to build lean mass and don't get enough protein from their diet. Whey protein is a left over product obtained from the production of cheese and up until a few years ago it was discarded as waste.

That was until a market was found for it and then it was marketed as a bodybuilding supplement. Keep in mind that eating more protein than the recommended daily dosage will not make you gain muscle faster.

But as long as your protein consumption is within the healthy boundaries of your program then you'll provide a healthy environment in your body that will promote lean mass gains.

Protein will also help keep your hunger in check as protein is very filling and not processed as quickly by the body as other macronutrients (like carbohydrates). A recent study done by a major university proved that women who consume high levels of protein in their diet are liker to lose weight faster than those who do not.

Omega-3 acids and fish oils

Omega 3 acids promote fat burning by switching on enzymes and proteins in your body that trigger fat-burning reactions in our body and fat cells. Omega 3 acids will also help muscle regenerate faster and are proven mood-enhancers which will help you avoid emotional eating by increasing the levels of serotonin and leptin signaling in your brain, which brings your appetite down and anxiety levels down as well.

Alli

A somewhat controversial pill that was originally created as the prescription drug Xenical which is now sold over the counter in a lower dose known as Alli. Alli prevents you from absorbing 25 percent of the fat that you get from aliments and it will definitely block some calorie absorption.

Alli can be consumed up to three times a day and a recent study proved that people who took Alli for six months lost around 50% more weight that those who didn't. Alli isn't entirely harmless though as it may cause loose stools and some diarrhea. Always check with your doctor before you start consuming any supplements.

HCA (Hydroxycitrate Acid)

HCA is a salt that is extracted from the brindal berry and the garcinia Cambodia. People in the Indian subcontinent have been using these salts for many years as a folk remedy to treat join and stomach ailments and can be found stateside as HCA or brindal berry and it helps you lose weight by reducing the amount of fat your body absorbs but also by increasing your metabolism and inhibit your appetite.

Glucomannan

Glucomannan extract is extracted from a south-Asian plant called Konjac which is high in fiber and is considered to be highly effective for diabetes and glucose control, but also offering weight-loss properties.

This plant has been for many years an important source of food for Asians and its high levels of fiber help absorb water in the GI tract, reducing the absorption of complex carbohydrates and LDL cholesterol and have been used for many years as a folk remedy for obesity.

Vitamin B

By getting a B-Complex vitamin you get the full range of vitamin B's including B1, B2, B3, B5, B6, B7, B9, and B12. Keep in mind that unless you have a notable b-vitamin deficiency you should limit the amount of B supplements you ingest. The most important out of all of these is by far B12 which helps bring energy levels up and increases the metabolism rate in your body, aiding with weight loss and fat absorption.

Chia Seeds

Chia seeds are fantastic for weight loss because they have high levels of Omega-3 and introduce a healthy way of introducing more omega-3 acids into your diet. Chia seeds also contain Lonolenic acid, a very important fatty acid that helps regulate fat-burning in the system. Since chia seeds do not have a distinctive taste or texture they can easily be incorporated into your diet by adding them into yogurt, oatmeal, smoothies, juices or other meals.

Coconut Oil

Usually considered one of the best "good fats" out there, you can incorporate coconut oil in your diet by substituting lard, canola or butter with Coconut oil which contains healthier saturated fats and even though coconut oil does have its fair share of detractors it has been proven to be a much healthier fat.

Chapter 32 - Motivation

Great, you've set your goals, you've planned your diet out and you've chosen an exercise regime. Now it is definitely time to get started... But you got your birthday coming up on Friday. And Saturday is pizza night and you definitely need to have a few beers on Sunday while watching the game, so you'll DEFINETELY start on Monday. Stop it.

We can all tell you're lying and that you'll never actually start. Maybe you'll tell your Facebook friends that you're eating right, or you'll instagram a few pictures on your first visit to the gym and then never come back. Stop it.

Being realistic about your faults as a human being is one of the most important steps when losing weight. We all lack motivation at one point or another, and it is easy to fall prey to junk food and back to your old habits, However with the right mindset and the right motivation you can easily find yourself eating right and working out because YOU ENJOY IT and not because you have to.

Approaching these lifestyles changes with the right mindset it is vital in order to make the changes that you so desperately want to make. Motivation plays a huge role in achieving this mindset. But, it is very important to understand what the right motivation is. Let's start off by not telling your Facebook friends that you're trying to lose weight. Yes, most people will motivate you and cheer you on.

But you have achieved nothing. Therefore since you have a (false) sense of accomplishment you will easily find yourself motivated to take a cheat day or to skip the gym that day. Having others ask you if you're losing weight or whether you've been working out feels AMAZING and I can guarantee that you will not want to skip the gym that day, it is truly one of the greatest feelings in the world!

Another thing to keep in mind is your long-term goals and permanent change in your behavior. If you go on a fad diet expecting short term amazing results you will most likely end up sorely disappointed.

Short term and fad diets are a recipe for failure because once you get off that diet guess what's going to happen? You're going to bounce right back. As soon as you return to your old eating habits the weight will come right back.

For permanent results you have to make permanent changes in your life, permanent changes in what you eat and permanent changes in your activity levels. Remember though! I don't want you walking your dog to the cornerstone and calling that a workout! I want you to sweat!

By setting a long-term goal and having it on your mind at all times you will find it easier to remember the changes that you need to make in order to achieve the goals you have set for yourself. Adapt to these new habits and adopt them. Think of soda as a special treat you can give to yourself every now and then and not as a staple on every food.

Think of dessert as something you get to have once or twice per month. Drink alcohol every day? You may have bigger problems. Seriously though, you'll know when something is right and when something is not. Be patient with yourself. Do not get discouraged. It will get easier over time. I guarantee it.

Do not use food as a coping mechanism. Sometimes we eat to comfort ourselves or to make ourselves feel better, some people use food as an escape mechanism or to avoid dealing with other issues in their lives. You need to look into the reasons why you eat and then find another way to deal with your feelings.

Go for a run, get into a hobby, go online and kill your enemies in a videogame, maybe try paintball? Whatever you decide to do to keep food off your mind is fine. Teach your brain to stop associating food with comfort. Remember, we eat to live; we do not live to eat.

It is okay to treat yourself to a snack every now and then but generally you HAVE to eat right and you HAVE to work out. You will hear a lot of bull on the internet from obese people who claim to be happy and who claim to be healthy. There's a huge movement going on right now, especially on the web of activism towards body acceptance and "Health at Every Size".

Nothing but a bunch of delusional obese people who have let their impulses control them and have to resort to finding a justification for their terrible habits and a community of equally deluded people who will do ANYTHING to justify their sad existence.

I can only hope that these people find how demented they are soon enough and make the changes they need to. For the time being we shouldn't worry about themselves as we're trying to improve ourselves and should not worry about what others say or do.

Going back to the topic of motivation though, it is important to see rethink the way you see weight loss. Don't turn it into a white or black situation where if you haven't achieved the goals you set for yourself then you have massively failed. Remember, THERE ARE NO SMALL VICTORIES when it comes to losing weight.

So you only lost 1 pound this week instead of the 2 you wanted to lose? Do not get discouraged. But also don't keep on doing the same thing and expecting the same results. Maybe try doing something a bit different; run an extra lap, drink skim milk instead of whole, maybe don't put cheese and mayo on your sandwiches?

Anyway, the idea is to make small changes that will amount to huge results later on. By finding small ways to improve your habits you will collectively achieve success in the long term.

This is why it is also hugely important to set realistic goals for yourself, do not set yourself up for failure, make sure you set sensible goals for yourself and stick to them. You're not going to be thin in 2 months.

You won't run a marathon by training for 4 weeks. Keep in mind that a sensible goal when losing weight is a maximum of 2 pounds per week. Any more than that and you'll be doing more harm than good. Also keep in mind that under any circumstances women should never eat less than 1400 calories per day and Men should generally never eat under 1800 calories (ideally 2000). Eat less than that and you're body will go into starvation mode.

Starvation mode is when your body realizes that it is not getting enough nutrients and tries to hold on to everything you have. See, your body uses glucose as a source of energy first. When glucose is depleted, the body then starts burning fat.

If you do not have enough energy to switch to fat-burning mode your body will get confused and try to hold on to everything that you've got. Including -yes- fat. This is why it is very important to never under eat when trying to lose weight. Remember, we're not trying to starve ourselves. We're just trying to lose a few pounds and get healthier while doing it. We do not wish to put our bodies at risk.

Also, take pictures! Take pictures of your body every week, in your undies, in the same mirror, same angle and same lighting as well. Nothing will motivate you more than seeing the actual results of your new habits. Weight yourself every day before you do ANYTHING. Get one of those iron beam scales if possible but if not then your bathroom scale will have to do.

Don't forget to reward yourself (obviously with non-food items). Maybe buy yourself a new book or that new album you've wanted for a few weeks. Treat yourself to a movie (easy on the popcorn though) or maybe buy a new computer mouse. I don't know.

Do whatever you have to do to keep yourself motivated to achieve your goals. Keep people with negative vibes away from you and do the same for people with unhealthy habits (I know it will be hard because sometimes even family members will try to keep you away from your goals) but stay strong, stay positive,

REMEMBER why you are doing this and think about how AMAZING you will look in 6 months, a year, two years, and five years. Think about all the looks you draw when you get into those jeans you've been dying to put on and that awesome strapless blouse you got as a gift that never fit quite right. It will feel amazing and the good thing is that you will become addicted to this filling, so you'll strive for more, you'll work out harder, you'll eat better, and you will go the extra mile to achieve the things that you want. Remember, if you want different results you will have to do things that you have never done. Losing weight it's simple (remember, calories in – calories out) but it is never easy.

Anyway, the idea is to keep yourself motivated to confront the little challenges that life will give you. As I mentioned before, no matter how strict you are with yourself, life will find a way to try to get you to cheat.

Office party, pizza nights, margarita Thursdays, your soap opera, the latest episode of that new reality show that is AMAZING (just kidding, no one really likes reality shows). But it is important that you stay strong and motivated. Keep in mind why it is that you're doing what you're doing.

Either endure the pain of discipline or endure the pain of regret. And believe me. Regret feels a thousand times worse. Nothing is worse than looking into the mirror and finding that you look terrible and hating who you have become. On the other hand, looking at yourself in the mirror and thinking "Damn, I look GREAT" will not only feed your ego but your soul as well. Nothing is better for motivation that self-appreciation for the new habits that you have acquired.

Finally, and I've decided to include this information under the motivation section because I know how hard it can be to drink enough water in a day. I used to HATE drinking water. I'm not sure why but I could easily go on for days without drinking water and living off coffee, diet soda, tea and other flavored substances.

But once you realize how important drinking water is it's something we all know is incredibly beneficial, yet most people do not drink nearly enough water. Stop what you're doing, and pour yourself a nice tall glass of crystal clear, refreshing water. Good. Feel better? Probably not but in the long term you will. You'll have better skin; your body will start to flush out toxins.

Drinking water will prevent your body from getting cramps and sprains. You'll improve your complexion and your bowel functions. You'll feel full faster. Get yourself a nice refillable bottle and stop spending so much money on disposable bottles (and polluting the planet as well) and refill it everywhere you go. There are drinking fountains and water coolers EVERYWHERE. If you work at an office you have no excuse, they usually have an endless supply of fresh, cool water for you to drink, so take your bottle with you and drink away!

You'll notice and improvement almost immediately and you'll be happy you decided to improve your current condition. I can guarantee that by increasing your activity levels, improving your diet, and drinking enough water you will lose weight! It is physically impossible not to!

Do not listen to those charlatans online who claim you will lose weight by tricking your body or by eating a bunch of salads. Do not fall for these tricks and motivate yourself to keep strong and healthy!

Chapter 33 - Things you'll notice as you're losing weight

Once you've figured out your caloric needs and stick to one of the programs describe in this book you'll start to notice significant changes. Not only in your body but in your mentality and habits as well. If you start to notice one or many of these things then that means you're on the right track for weight loss.

Clothes fitting better

One of the first and most obvious signs of weight loss for most people. Remember those pants you haven't been able to get into for the last 5 years? You'll notice you can comfortably slide in and out of them quite comfortably without struggling to button that button or to bring that zipper up. This brings us to our next point...

Needing to wear a belt

Or to punch out a new hole in your belt in order to keep those pants up! While this may seem like a nuisance to most people, the feeling you get when you know you have to get a new belt is simply fantastic, you won't even care! And as for your old belt. Either throw it away or give it to someone else. You won't need it ever again.

Feeling healthier

Remember how you felt every time you had to climb that dreaded set of stairs at work? Now you can breeze through them without breaking a sweat or feeling like you're going to pass out. Same feeling applies to simple tasks that represented a challenge before like walking to your car or getting out of bed. If you feel more flexible and thinner then you probably are!

Thinking twice about eating empty calories

Before you made healthy changes in your life you wouldn't think twice about eating a whole pint of ice cream or half a pizza. But now that you have made a conscious decision to change your life you'll think twice before eating junk like this. Maybe you'll settle for a scoop of ice cream instead of the whole pint or for a few chips instead of the whole bag.

Becoming better in bed

It is not a secret that changing your unhealthy habits will give you more flexibility and endurance in bed. Not only will you notice these changes when it comes but performing... but you'll also notice that you've become more confident and this will definitely reflect when it comes to pleasing your partner. Don't be surprised by loud clapping and fanfare after you're done.

Having more energy

By far, one of the most encouraging aspects of losing weight and getting healthier is discovering your levels of energy have come up. You won't lose your breath or steam as quickly, your day will last you longer, you'll be able to achieve more and less time and to do things you weren't able to do before. Like dropping to the ground into a full squat. You'll find yourself pumped to do things you haven't done before. You'll wake up wanting to do things like a hundred pushups or go out for a run.

Muscle definition

We have talked about this before but I'll go ahead and talk about it again. As your body fat percentages come down, your muscle definition will improve, whether you have small or large muscles you will inevitably look better. Don't get discouraged if you don't see anything in the abdominal region as this is where we store most of our fat. You'll have to work out a lot harder if you want to see definition in this area. It is definitely not impossible, so as long as you stick to your program and keep achieving your goals you will eventually rock that six pack!

You'll get more compliments

People will stare at you (in a good way though). Nothing feels better than having someone admire your physique (especially if it's an equally attractive person) and since you'll have improved confidence as well you'll know how to react to these situations without looking like a fool! People will treat you with more respect, they'll listen to what you have to say and admire you for the person you have become.

Your face will look a lot better

One of the first things that people will notice when you lose weight is how thin your face will look after dropping a few pounds. For some reason our chins and our cheeks are one of the first place where fat seems to go away quicker so even by dropping 5-10 pounds your face will look significantly slimmer. You'll look better in headshots and selfish and you'll love the new "you". This is why it is important to praise yourself for progress (no matter how small it may be).

Your skin will get better, you'll smell better too

I'm sure there's a scientific principle behind this; I'm just not too sure what it is. But when people lose weight their skin will get better, you'll have this natural shine to you that people will notice. You will no longer look like a chicken a rotisserie and your natural body odor will improve as well.

Of course, using a decent deodorant and some good cologne will go a long ways towards improving your overall presence but you will naturally look and feel better without needing a lot of help from beauty products.

You'll find yourself motivated to achieve greater things

Success is the most addicting drug out there. Once you achieve a tiny little bit of success you will never be able to stop there. You'll end up wanting more and more. You'll want to lose more weight, you'll want to set a new personal record at the gym, and you'll want to do one more rep, one more set. You'll never be able to stop now. Success is one hell of a drug and people crave it like no other. You'll find yourself motivated to always strive for more and to never settle.

One final thing and something that I believe is very important. Have you ever heard the phrase "surround yourself with winners"? What does this mean? Well it is actually very simple, it means that if you want to become a winner you must surround yourself with winners.

Whether it is to learn something new or to copy their winning habits it ends up being true in the long term. When losing weight and getting healthier you must surround yourself with people who will make you want to get healthy. As I Said before there are people who will try to bring you down.

To try "just a tiny slice of cake" or just a "small slice of pizza". I'm not telling you to avoid them completely from now on. But do not let yourself to be dragged down by their unhealthy habits and negative views on life. Avoid drinking. Avoid smoking; surround yourself with winners, people who enjoy going out for a morning run at 5 am before work.

People who will hit the gym at 10 at night because that's the only time they can go. Go to your gym on a Friday night and talk to the people there. The people there are people who truly love what they do. They don't care that it's a Friday or that it's late. They are going to do what they want to do not let themselves get anxious by what society dictates.

Chapter 34 - Conclusion

Let's go back a bit so we can understand what I've been trying to explain to you in this book. The conscious decisions you make in your life will ultimately determine whether you succeed or fail in your weight-losing efforts. You can continue with your terrible habits and do a bit of exercise here and there and expect to be successful but we all know that will not happen.

It is important to be aware of your limitations and your goals, keep a strong will and stick to what you have planned out.

Remember the basic formula for weight loss we discussed in the first pages of this book? Calories in minus calories out. You create a caloric deficit and you will lose weight. Remember, it is science and a law of thermodynamics.

However, it is important to remember that losing weight does not automatically mean you're healthier. Yes, it is a very important step in achieving your goals but it is not the only step you will need to take. Healthiness comes from within, and thus it is vital to remember that your must also exercise.

Dieting only will not cut it; you need to achieve greater things like more endurance, more strength, and more flexibility. Become a better human being and aim to improve yourself every day. Do not let others discourage you. Do not do things to please others, but do them to please yourself and to satisfy your expectations.

I hope that the changes that you have decided to make are permanent and that you stick with them for the rest of your life. Remember, it is not only important to live a long life but to live a quality life. Wouldn't you like to chase your grandkids on food through hills and streets rather than have to watch them seated in and old scooter?

Your habits will ultimately mark your success or failure in life. This is why I recommend giving up any nasty habits that you have picked up along the way. I'm talking about things like smoking cigarettes or drinking. I'm not saying I don't enjoy a neat glass of scotch every once in a while.

But I use it to motivate myself only and I don't let it become a crutch. Don't be that guy or girl that downs a six pack of beer every night before bed to help you "go to sleep". You know what else put you to sleep? A good 3 mile run and a warm shower. You'll sleep like a baby without ingesting empty calories and you'll get rid of that ugly beer-belly.

I hope you have enjoyed the advice in this book and even if it helps you just a tiny little bit in achieving your goals then I'll be satisfied. Thank you for taking the time to read my book and Good luck to you!

Chapter 35 - ACCESS TO BONUS VIDEO AND RECIPES

First of all, we'd like to give you a **BIG HEARTY** Thank you for purchasing our book. We strive to offer you the best service possible and certainly hope that we've been able to give you some kind of ***VALUE for your money's worth!***

If you've learned anything or got at least **1 GOOD IDEA** from our book, we kindly ask that you share that with us and leave some feedback.

Your humble feedback will not only help us to push forward with more helpful products to serve you better, but will also help other lovely customers (such as yourself) to make a purchasing decision as each review will be online for **ALL TO SEE!**

Once Again We Thank You for Your Time with Us and We Wish You **GREAT SUCCESS ON YOUR JOURNEY!**

(Just Click on the Link Below or Copy and Enter It in Your URL, then Copy and Paste the Password in the Box)

http://videoreviewteam.com/flat-belly-miracle

Password: flatbelly123

NOTE: Also If you want ***MORE IN DEPTH LESSONS*** on *How You Can Lose Belly Fat* (There is a Link at the Bottom of the Videos Page) ...**Thank You Once Again!**

www.ingramcontent.com/pod-product-compliance
Lightning Source LLC
Chambersburg PA
CBHW070237290526
45789CB00004B/1655